A Girl's Guide to Femdom

*Tips, Tricks, Punishments and Rituals
for Every Day of the Year*

Lucy Fairbourne

Published by Velluminous Press
www.velluminous.com

ISBN-13: 978-1-905605-51-4

1.0

A Girl's Guide to Femdom

*Tips, Tricks, Punishments and Rituals
for Every Day of the Year*

Lucy Fairbourne

Contents

Introduction

This book is intended for the woman who has embarked on a femdom-oriented relationship with her man, and who is hungry for some empowering, kinky and fun scenarios to explore with him. If that describes you, welcome!

If you're not yet ready for actual scenarios — if this all seems very strange and puzzling to you — may I suggest turning to one of my introductory femdom books before diving in to the rest of this one.

Take Care, Not Risks ...

This book is intended for responsible, consenting adults.

It contains scenarios and ideas related to a way of loving that includes safe and consensual discipline administered by a caring Mistress to her willing slave. If you're not sure where your man's personal boundaries are, talk things through in advance and arrange a safe-word that he can use to call a halt if things get too much.

Do not proceed with any activity until you are sure it is safe, sane and consensual.

... and Take Care of Yourself, Too!

The ideas in this book are suggestions. There's never any need for you to do anything you're uncomfortable with or to go further than you desire. Don't allow your submissive partner to pressure you into activities you don't enjoy. In the long run, that can't work for either of you.

January - February: Weeks 1-5

Week 1: Punishment Tokens

You will need two types of coin-like token.

You can easily find these for sale online; gambling chips or gaming tokens (including antique or historical ones, if you'd like something a bit different) are ideal. If you wish, get your submissive man to do the research and purchasing leg-work — subject to your final approval, of course!

Designate one style of token for reward and one for punishment. If you can, make the choice symbolic — gold- or silver-colored tokens for rewards, perhaps, and plainer-looking ones for punishment.

Keep a supply of tokens about your person and hand him rewards and punishments as appropriate. Or, if you'd like it to be a surprise, quietly slip one into his pocket.

If appropriate, explain what he did to earn each punishment token (unless it ought to be obvious). He is to remember the infraction and enter it into the Punishment Book later. Each token whose cause he can't remember counts as an extra infraction.

At the end of each week (or other period) make him account for his tokens before returning them to you, and Reward or Punish him as appropriate.

If he ends up with more punishment than reward tokens at the end of the period, assign him an extra punishment. As time goes on, you may adjust this so that he has to work harder to avoid punishment in future weeks. For example, inform him that you expect him to have at least two more reward tokens than punishment tokens.

Week 2: Bath Slave

Instruct him to run you a bath. He should add your preferred kind of bubbles or bath salts, check the water temperature, light candles, make everything as you like it. He is to place a small bell at the side of the bath. Make sure he has the information and materials he needs to prepare everything properly.

While you are preparing to enter the bath he is to choose your fluffiest bath towel, setting it to warm if necessary.

Tell him that you expect him to meet you with the warm towel as you emerge from the bath, but in the meantime he is to go off to attend to some secondary chore that you consider important. Explain the punishment he faces if he disappoints you in any way. Make it something he would prefer to avoid. Since this is a bathroom scenario, how about a cold shower? Or perhaps being assigned to scrub the bathroom until everything sparkles? Or, give him the choice ... and then decide whether to go along with his request or to compel him into accepting the alternative anyway.

When you have soaked for long enough, ring for him if he's not already there. The fact that you had to ring means that he was not attentive enough, so a punishment will be due. He may also earn a punishment if he did not complete the secondary chore to your satisfaction. The final way he can earn a punishment is by disturbing you through intrusive checking or by arriving too early with the towel.

If he manages everything gracefully and in a timely manner, consider rewarding him.

Note: because of the time element, this is a difficult task. You will achieve maximum erotic tension by making it seem challenging but possible, so help him out if you wish by providing some clues or cooperation:

- Leave the bathroom door ajar so that he can unobtrusively check on you.

- Assign a secondary chore that is not too demanding and that can be frequently interrupted.
- Help him out by listening for his approach and adjusting your timing, as long as he's reasonably close to what you wanted.
- Play some soft, relaxing music of suitable duration as you soak, so that by listening carefully he can judge when it's about to end.
- Order him to figure out a way of safely monitoring the water temperature from elsewhere in your home (temperature monitors are available for hot tubs and pools) so he can judge when your bath is cooling off. If he starts relaxing and taking things too much for granted, toy with him by removing the sensor from the hot water.

As suggested above, you might sometimes choose to be capricious and to make the task difficult or impossible (it should seem possible to him as he goes about his business; the fact that you've decided to make things more than usually challenging is your little secret). It can be more fun for both of you, if you behave slightly differently from time to time.

Week 3: Telephone Service

When you call an open-minded and trusted girlfriend, have him make the call on your behalf, as if he were your secretary or personal assistant. He has to greet your friend politely and explain that you have told him to call her before handing the phone to you.

Obviously, you need to be sure that the recipient of the call is not going to be freaked out by this!

If this doesn't seem challenging enough, consider pushing him further. Maybe have him remove some or all of his clothes before making the call; once he's conveniently exposed you should find it easy perform some stimulating and distracting activity of your choice, while he tries to carry out his conversation ...

Week 4: *The Language of t*

Train him to respond to signals from your pre
correction as he goes down on you. Choose s
controllable; a riding crop works well once yo
with its use. Keep the signals simple, since you w   ιο dis-
tract yourself by remembering complex sequences.
For example:

- one sharp stroke = slow down, take your time
- two strokes = pick up the pace
- three strokes = finish me off now.

He might hope for more guidance than you can comfortably
give while enjoying him, so keep it as simple as you need. The language of *"Strike"* = *"Go Faster"* is natural enough to be used with
very little effort or distraction at all.

Week 5: *In Vino Veritas*

Have him pour you a big glass of your favorite wine. He should also
prepare a selection of small, tasty treats for you while providing
himself with a bottle of water.

Have him strip, then tie him face-up and spread-eagled on the
bed. Straddle him while you blindfold him. If you like, take the opportunity to tease him in any way you choose, but don't allow him
to get very far.

Now stimulate his naked skin with various objects. For example: a feather, a silk scarf, the wet stem of one of the flowers he
brought you, the point of a knitting needle, your finger nail, the end
of your riding crop, a make-up brush, a hair brush, your hair, different parts of a high-heeled shoe. Use ice or hot candle-wax if you're
into that kind of play; these will be easy for him to identify but the
ability to inflict intense, surprising sensations is worth it.

His only task is to guess what you are using.

If he guesses wrong, he gets a slow dribble of water from the water bottle (choose one with a sports top, since controlling the flow of water into his mouth might not be easy while he's spread-eagled on the bed. If you prefer more contact than that, take a sip of water yourself and kiss it into his mouth. Or, if you're in the mood and feeling kind, straddle him again and let him fleetingly taste your pussy instead.

After three wrong guesses, move to the next object, but assign him a stroke of your palm, paddle or riding crop as a punishment to be delivered when he's no longer tied on his back — assuming you prefer to punish his posterior.

If he guesses correctly, reward him by allowing him one of your tasty morsels and/or by kissing a sip of wine into his mouth. If he guesses particularly quickly, consider substituting the superior reward of a more intense (but still fleeting) pussy-tasting. Then move to a different object.

When you've run out of objects, complete his reward by allowing him to orally pleasure you.

February - March: Weeks 6-9

Week 6: Punishment Book

Acquire (or have your slave acquire) a suitable blank journal in which infractions and punishments can be recorded. Ideally the journal will be handsome and imposing, perhaps with a leather binding and high-quality paper to reflect the ritual power it will come to contain.

Create rituals surrounding the book. For example:

- Where will it be stored?
- Will it be under lock and key?
- Who must/may access it?
- Who will enter punishments that are due? (this could be your slave's responsibility, if you prefer)
- Will a particular kind of pen and/or ink be used?
- Who will mark off punishments that have been completed?
- If your slave is not allowed to consult the book himself, will you instead have him ritually fetch it when you wish to use it?
- If your slave is to consult the book, under what circumstances is this permitted? Supervised? Unsupervised? Only by the light of the Punishment Candle?

If you fill up the punishment book, set it aside as a permanent record and start another.

Week 7: Reclining with Grapes

Have him kneeling while you recline. He should be naked; you may start out lightly dressed if you wish.

He is to peel grapes from a well-chilled bunch and feed them to you. The discarded skins go into a bowl; you may underline his status by feeding him one of these from time to time. Optionally feed him whole grapes too, unless you have decided to deepen the sense of degration he feels by limiting him to the skins.

From time to time, take a peeled grape from him, push it between your toes, and have him eat it from there. He is to lick up juices that end up on your skin, too.

If he deserves more intimacy than that, squeeze a grape onto your breasts, or let him take one from your mouth, or allow him to eat a few grapes off your pussy (it's not a good idea to actually insert grapes, or indeed most foods, into your vagina. The idea is to have fun, not a yeast infection!).

Grapes are ideal because once peeled they are a bit messy and have edible skins, but other fruit such as segments of sweet citrus will also work, if you prefer them.

When you are ready, signal that he is to go down on you.

Week 8: Timed Masturbation

This one works best if your man has developed the expectation that you will provide all his orgasms when you're together, or if he feels some embarrassment about touching himself in front of you, but at a level that he is able to overcome in his desire to please you.

On the other hand, if he's a sexual exhibitionist who gets turned on by performing for you, it may be all too easy for him to comply. If that's the case, spice things up a little with one of the variations below.

Set a timer and order him to masturbate to completion before it rings, while you settle down to enjoy the show. Use comments and commands to create a more dominant and brazen mood, or watch quietly if you prefer.

If he fails to climax in time, he doesn't get to come ... for the next week (or whatever period you determine).

Variation 1: set two timers a short period apart; he has to come during the interval between the first and second timer going off.

Variation 2: proceed as normal but as he's getting close, order him to stop and to please you with his mouth instead.

If he doesn't seem to be coping well with this game (for example, if he cannot get hard or cannot get anywhere near climax) then he may have deeper issues about performing in front of you. Bear in mind that this shyness will not be something he has chosen, so keep things light and playful; maybe oil up your hands and take over the stimulation that he can't manage for himself. Later, talk things over so you'll know how (and whether) to approach the subject in future. Only you and he together can judge how best to proceed.

Week 9: Strip Jack Naked

Play strip poker, or any game you both enjoy where losing a hand or round can translate into losing clothes. Whoever ends up naked first is the loser, at which point the winner gets to choose an erotic forfeit that the loser must pay.

If he loses a point, he must strip off an item of clothing as usual. Once one of his garments is gone, it stays gone.

If you lose a point, you may remove clothing if you wish, but you may also "borrow back" your discarded clothes.

Every time you "borrow back", mark down a forfeit (of your choice) that he must pay. Ask his opinion about what forfeit is appropriate if you wish, but you are the one who decides.

Clearly, you are going to win unless you actively choose to lose and submit yourself to his forfeit (there's no harm in that, once in a while, right? It's entirely up to you!) Once you have won the final game, have him settle his forfeits.

March - April: Weeks 10-13

Week 10: Beast of Burden

When you're out shopping together, treat him as your personal beast of burden by giving him your heavy stuff to carry. There's no need to ask his permission; just give him your bags or parcels, or place your items into the bag he is already carrying.

Don't show any gratitude, or concern about whether he can manage (within reason); a consensual male slave wants to be strong enough to serve his Mistress's in any way she pleases. When you act on the unacknowledged assumption that he is strong enough, then you are flattering his male ego as well as giving him the submissive reward of being valuable to you.

Of course, you need to keep an eye out to see if he really does need help — you could open the car for him when you get back to it, for example, or help him to stow parcels securely on public transport. The heavy lifting is for him, though, and he is expected to thank you for any help you offer.

Once you and he arrive back home, feel free to acknowledge that you enjoyed taking advantage of him in this way.

Week 11: A Week in Chastity

Tell him he isn't permitted to climax for a week (or however long you choose; make it long enough to challenge him but not excessively long — think days or weeks, rather than months). If you're not sure how long to say, just tell him he's not allowed to climax until you give permission, which will depend on his good behavior. Then you can decide on the end date later, as you learn how you and he respond to this experience.

During this period of chastity, the only orgasms he is to experience will be the ones he gives you, or watches you giving yourself if you choose to indulge him in that way. Try tying him up while you masturbate in front of him, to prevent him from taking matters into his own hands. Even if you trust him to behave in that regard, placing him under physical restraint is a powerful demonstration of your loving authority. Enjoying a "substitute penis" in the form of a dildo or vibrator also sends a message, and one that may hold even more erotic power for your submissive man.

Subject him to regular teasing sessions where you stroke and stimulate him without permitting him to come. Such "prick teasing" may seem cruel and even unbearable to him, but it will also be intensely pleasurable; the longer he is denied release, the more he will need your teasing touch.

You may well find that he becomes more intensely submissive than usual after a period of frustration. Even if you don't insist on specific periods of chastity, taking control of his orgasms and limiting them to a level where he remains constantly horny around you, can only make him more susceptible to your female power. If you enjoy holding that power that his chastity gave you, reward him by letting him know as well as with physical teasing.

Many couples find that male chastity is "femdom rocket fuel", since it builds up the male libido (a potent force!) in the service of the female, and in a way that can be directed and controlled by her. If you and your man enjoy that aspect of the activity, think about getting a chastity device so that you can lock him up more securely. Even if you trust him not to cheat, or if it's impractical for him to wear the device long-term, the ability to have him locked up so intimately while you have the only key, offers an intensity of control that goes beyond his "promise to behave" — no matter how earnestly that promise is meant.

Week 12: Oral Inspection

This is all about communicating the femdom fact that his mouth is your property. When you permit him to serve you orally, it is you granting him a favor and not the other way around. You can underscore this by having him cleanse and purify his mouth before being permitted to approach his Mistress.

Establish rituals such as:

- Pre-worship mouth inspection. Be as intrusive as you like. Use a suitable gag if you wish (see below). Make him open wide and hold it while you manipulate his jaw, inspect his teeth and generally invade him with your fingers. Make like you're a buyer at a horse auction and he's the beast you're considering.
- Make it clear that you consider his mouth to be yours, and that you are naturally interested in how well he is keeping it on your behalf.
- Before any occasion where you might permit or demand cunnilingus, have him brush, rinse with mouthwash, etc. before he approaches your pussy.
- While you're at it, why not check his beard area too? You're entitled to stubble-free service.
- If you have him perform other oral activities such as anilingus or foot-worship, the same rituals apply; every part of your body is just as sacred as your pussy, and deserving of the same reverence.

Variation: Make love or engage in femdom play while his mouth is stopped with a suitable gag.

Things to try:

- your panties or other underwear
- a ball gag
- a bit gag (like the bit used in a horse's bridle)
- a dildo gag (see Dildo Play)
- an 'O' ring gag where he can't close his mouth
- a medical style gag used to keep the mouth held open for full access or inspection (look for a "Jennings Gag")
- make him hold your riding crop in his mouth while waiting to be punished, or while you spank or paddle him with something else.

Week 13: The Punishment Candle

This is a special candle that is only lit during formal corporal punishment sessions, typically ones that occur in your bedroom. Linking the lighting of the candle and the formal punishment of your slave — ensuring that one never happens without the other — can create a highly erotic ritual association. The use of a punishment candle fits in very well if you already enjoy using this intimate form of illumination during your femdom scenes … and if you don't, give it a try!

Establish rituals around the use of the candle. For example:

- Keep a special lighter or matchbox for lighting the punishment candle; do not allow the lighter/matchbox to be used for anything else.
- Keep the candle locked away with other ritual items such as your whips or the Punishment Book.
- Always light the punishment candle first, then use that candle to light any other candles that will be used to illuminate the planned scene.

- When the punishment candle has burned down to a stub, use it to light the replacement so that the flame's lineage and essence is preserved.
- Have your man make the punishment candles (have him research candle-making if necessary), incorporating the wax from previous candles into each new one.
- If you use hot-wax play, you could use the punishment candle itself, or light the hot-wax candle from the punishment candle. Decide which, and make it a consistent ritual.

April - May: Weeks 14-17

Week 14: Foot-bath and Pedicure

Have him give you a luxurious foot bath, with a towel spread before the couch, a large bowl of water at just the right temperature, and your favorite brand of bubbles or other product. Let him take his time about servicing you, then let him dry you off.

When he's done with the foot bath, have him give you whatever pedicure services you require. He may require instruction and practice before he becomes competent at this, so allow him time to learn — but also recognise that his male inexperience can provide opportunities for "training" and punishment!

If you decide he deserves a reward, permit him to massage your feet with the oil of your choice.
Then have him kiss them, if you so desire. If you're in the mood for it, have him work his way up from there.

Boost the dominance-submission dynamic by having a riding crop to hand during the whole process, and by controlling his (lack of) clothing as he kneels before you. The riding crop won't be of much use while he's working on your feet, but it might come into its own later on…

Week 15: Sex Toy Inventor

Make him devise a kinky sex toy intended to please you.

It should be something of an appropriate level for his skills.
If it pleases you, use it. If it's not, make him pay for something that will.

Here is a simple suggestion in case he's a complete beginner at this type of thing: have him make a unique leather collar, whip, or other toy. Almost anyone should be able to make a workable collar or punishment strap from an old leather belt. If necessary, your man should research methods, tools and materials. Obviously, if a simple project wouldn't challenge him enough, then suggest (or get him to suggest) something more complicated.

He is only to present his creation to you when he is confident about its quality and finish (including the oiling, waxing or polishing of any natural materials such as wood or leather). If you're happy with it, show him by accepting and using his offering. If not, give him a playful punishment and instruct him to do the work again.

Week 16: Reward and Punishment

A well-known paradox within femdom-based relationships occurs because the submissive male wants to be punished, and may therefore misbehave in order to get that desire fulfilled. As a dominant female you would obviously prefer obedience from your man, so how do you deal with the risk that by punishing him, you might be encouraging him to provoke more of the same?

One approach is to choose punishments that he finds unpleasant — a cold shower, for example, or perhaps a tedious household chore that he must do alone without the benefit of your erotic attention (which is what he is really after, when seeking a femdom punishment).

Another way is to actively use punishment as a reward, not just as a deterrent. To do this, you must become aware of the difference between punishment that you inflict as part of your female right to correct him, and punishment that you offer because your man desires it. Only the presentation need differ:

"I am going to whip you because last time we were together, you came before you had permission. Let it be a lesson to you."

"I am going to whip you because you pleased me so well that I want to fix the occasion in your mind to help you repeat it next time."

That way, he knows he can earn the desired punishment by doing the right thing, and the incentive for him to misbehave is diminished. The physical sensation of the whipping might be virtually identical in each case, but how you and he feel about it will be very different.

Week 17: Sauce for the Goose

This game is about erotically demonstrating your female superiority and contrasting it your man's lowly status. If your man has a foot-fetish, it can also be used to indulge his passion for your feet.

For however long you choose, he will only be entitled to be pleased by your hands (and optionally by your feet). You will be receiving pleasure from his mouth, his hands, a dildo, a vibrator, a strap-on that he wears; anything except his penis.

The hand-jobs you provide will be strictly limited to what you wish to give; the attentions he offers in return will be unstinting.

When you decide to give him a hand-job, arrange him on his back. For maximum control, tie his hands to the headboard of the bed. Enjoy his mouth while you have him like that, if you wish.

When it's his turn, use your preferred oil or lube and go to town. You can demand that he asks Permission to Come if you like, or incorporate other games such as Sexy Scrunchies.

If you enjoy foot-play, arrange yourself so you can stretch one leg out onto his body. Put your foot on his chest to show that you have "vanquished" him. For even more intensity, move it up to pin him by the throat. Or, push the sole of your foot onto his face, then slip your toes into his mouth.

If you use your feet to stimulate his penis, they will get messed up by oil and pre-cum. Have him lick them clean (use an edible lube!) if you wish. If you have gotten semen on them, his submissiveness will be ebbing along with his satisfied libido, but you might still be able to persuade him to lick that clean, too…

May - June: Weeks 18-22

Week 18: Countdown to Climax

This is a good scenario to play out once you start exploring male chastity.

Take your man to bed and begin to make love normally, ensuring that you receive plenty of oral stimulation as part of your foreplay. When you move to intercourse, inform him that he is only allowed a certain number of strokes; he is expected to make you come within that limit. Choosing the number of strokes is a balance between satisfying your own needs while leaving your slave feeling disappointed (and submissively aroused at the same time) when he hears how little he is to be allowed.

The power and control that you get from being on top is ideal in this scenario, but do whatever you find more comfortable, while bearing in mind that the only orgasm being planned here is yours. Avoid anything that risks an unplanned ejaculation.

Depending on the outcome of the limited number of strokes, assign him a suitable reward or punishment:

- If you come precisely on the final stroke, he's allowed a (non-orgasmic) reward, such as worshipping you orally once you desire this service.
- If you come before the end of the count, either allow him to enjoy the strokes you promised or (if you prefer to stop or suspect he might ejaculate) then indulge his need for erotic cruelty by cutting things short.
- If you don't come within the count, then make him stop and satisfy you with his mouth instead, or in whatever other way you prefer...
- ...or allow him to continue intercourse until you climax, but punish him for the extra strokes he "stole".

Week 19: Naked in the Kitchen.

Make him cook for you, undressed except for accoutrements such as a slave collar if you use one on him.

He's permitted to wear whatever covering is needed to protect from heat, spills, splashes etc. (oven gloves and an apron, for example), otherwise he should be essentially nude.

Go into the kitchen from time to time to observe and assess his work. Grade him on the final meal, too. Consider different aspects such as presentation, timeliness, the quality of various dishes, the attentiveness of service.

If he is permitted to eat with you, assign him the less perfect portion if there is one. For example, if an egg is broken or a steak is overcooked, that should be on his plate rather than yours.

If he serves something particularly delicious, express your appreciation and allow him a suitable reward.

Week 20: Waiter Service

As part of the previous scenario, or any time you are dining at home, have him wait at your table instead of eating with you.

Decide how he is to be dressed while he does this, and let him know.

He is to bring your food, serve your drinks, clear away courses and bring the new ones. If wine is an important part of your lives, have him act as your sommelier while letting him know you will be judging him on the quality of his wine suggestions and how well they match the food being served.

Assess other aspects of presentation and performance, too.

If you'd like to spice up your dining experience, create the fantasy that you're in a busy restaurant. Tell your waiter you are an important restaurant critic and his job is on the line if he doesn't take special care of you, even though there are many other tables demanding his attention. Make the scandalous suggestion that he is to get beneath the table to attend to your tired feet or to service you orally. Naturally, he has no choice but to obey…

Once your waiter has finished serving you, you may wish to tip him with Punishment/Reward Tokens.

Week 21: Strict Wife's Domestic Servant

Order him to assist you with chores that are easier with two. For example, cleaning the floors (he can move heavy furniture so you can clean beneath it) or changing the sheets.

The idea is more about getting him work smoothly with you, and to learn your ways while having some femdom fun, than about reducing your workload … after all, if that was your main goal you could just have your man do it all on his own.

Encourage him to be a good servant by anticipating your needs. A submissive male should be eager to please his Mistress in this regard and might perform surprisingly well, but push him hard anyway; that is part of the game.

If you plan to physically punish him on the spot for shortcomings (recommended) then it's best if he's naked or under-dressed while he works, since clothes will protect him and make him feel less vulnerable.

With time and practice, he should become better at anticipating your needs, and you may need to raise the standards you demand of him to create further excuses for punishment.

This scenario is not necessarily an efficient way of actually getting the chores done!

Week 22: Timed Massage

Have him massage you in any way you wish, but set a timer to determine the duration.

Don't be scared of setting up an extended massage. This is about your pleasure and relaxation, and his servitude and sacrifice.

Don't tolerate any loss of concentration or force as his hands get tired. Be strict if necessary.

When the timer goes off, he should stop but wait to see if you re-set it. If so then he is to begin again.

Boost the dominance-submission dynamic by controlling his (lack of) clothing while he massages you.

At the end, reward good service by expressing your appreciation. If he is conveniently naked, consider emphasising your satisfaction with him by repaying the massage strokes he has given you with a few Rewarding Strokes of your strap or riding crop, before you allow him to get dressed.

Variation: if you enjoy receiving extended, leisurely oral attention, use the same timing technique to indulge yourself in that way, too.

Whether you are receiving a relaxing massage or erotic pleasure, be prepared to communicate your preferences and needs firmly and clearly; a truly submissive man will be far more interested in whatever guidance you can offer in how best to please you, than he is about having his male ego flattered with false praise.

June - July: Weeks 23-26

Week 23: Role Reversal

When you are out together (or in company, if you are confident and brave) reverse the traditional gender roles.

In fact, go further than that. Consider how the relations between men and women would have been in the 1950s or 1960s, and reverse that.

For example, the man would almost always have been the car-owner and would have automatically driven to the date. Assuming you enjoy driving too, you can turn that on its head. That's particularly effective if you and he have slipped into the old model where "the guy always drives."

(He can be the one who stays sober in order to drive home, if you like. At one time and in some company, it was generally the woman who was expected to do that).

In the restaurant, order his food for him (choose it too, if you wish). Order the wine or other drinks. Take the lead when it comes to dealing with the waiter; inform your man that he is to defer to your interactions. When the meal is finished, make sure you receive the check and hand the payment over.

If you need to purchase or pick up movie- or show-tickets in person, be the one who deals with the theater representative.

Depending on where you are and who you're with, explicit role-reversal may cause some raised eyebrows. Not every friend or relative is understanding or open-minded and not every couple who enjoys femdom play is immune to embarrassment, so use your discretion.

Feel free to push things in the other direction if it's more convenient or more fun. For example, while a 1950s guy would have opened the car door for his girl, you can still have your man do that for you. Or, if you'd prefer to relax while your man stands in line for tickets, stay with the traditional gender role where he would have been the one expected to do just that.

Week 24: Strong but Submissive

Being in a female-led relationship is empowering, but power brings responsibility too. What if you feel that too much of the erotic responsibility in your relationship has ended up with you, and not enough with him?

An obvious answer is that you are empowered to shift some of that responsibility back to him.

So, if your man's submissive nature makes him a little more passive in the bedroom that you'd prefer, give him "standing orders" that he is to take the lead in pleasing you.

For example, tell him he's expected to try to seduce you every night (or however often you prefer) before you both sleep.
If you respond by saying "No", or "We'll do something else" then he is expected to comply immediately. You are still in control; you've delegated some of your power but you are entitled to take it back at any instant.

Alternatively, you can leave the control with him. Just lie back and experience every detail of what he has in mind for you and for himself … or you can let things proceed to your own satisfaction and then tell him "goodnight," at which point he has to stop no matter how horny he is feeling.

Or, take things to the point where he's sure he's about to get lucky. Maybe he will! If you decide that he's not, then you're playing a simple male chastity game where you've led him on before cutting him off. Most guys would resent this kind of "Teasing and Denial". A submissive man (particularly one who has the male chastity kink) might hate the frustration, but he'll also love the fact that you caused it and that he's powerless to do anything about it.

Week 25: Sexy Writer

Have him write you a sexy story or poem.

Give him a character, setting, theme or other direction if you like.

Either let him write it in his own time and in his own way, or place him clearly in his slave-role by controlling how he is clothed, where he sits, and what writing tools or instruments he uses. If you wish to increase the pressure further, set a reasonable time limit.

If you and he enjoy school-Mistress fantasies, correct the finished work as if you were his teacher (you can even use red ink if you like!) Or, incorporate it into the Class Action scenario.

Punish/reward according to the effort he made, as much as by the results. As a caring Mistress demanding and then assessing your man's creative and self-revealing effort, you will wish to keep any criticism playful and/or constructive rather than belittling.

If the story has enough erotic power, consider offering the unique reward of acting out one of its key scenes with him.

Week 26: Shaving, Plucking, Waxing

Decide how much hair he's allowed, and enforce your decision.

Your man's body hair is a sign of his masculinity; removing it is a powerful symbol of his subjection to your female power. It can also make him feel more sensitive and more vulnerable "down there". Experiment with cropping/shaving his head hair too, if you like.

Depending on how far you want him to go and how intimately involved you wish to be, you could:

- actively participate in the depilation
- perform regular inspections to make sure he is complying with your instructions

- if he is liable to go further than you wish, set limits about what he is allowed to remove
- inspect only occasionally, for example at the beginning of a scene where he is naked and exposed.

Use your own preference and (as always) your common sense, and be flexible about what he is to do. For example, if shaving causes ingrown hairs and/or an excessively bristly feel, maybe allow him to trim closely with guarded hair clippers instead.

It should go without saying that any depilation tool or product used on the genitals or other sensitive skin, must be safe for that use. You or he must always check the instructions carefully and test a small area first.

There's no reason why your man should have all the depilation fun, so if you don't already do so, consider removing or trimming your own pubic hair too, in whatever way is most comfortable for you. Once you've experienced his tongue on your bare pussy, you might never go back.

July - August: Weeks 27-31

Week 27: Responding to the Whip

This is a kind of time-out from the normal Mistress-slave scenario, one where you will work together to deepen your bond of mutual knowledge and trust.

Schedule a discipline session that is neither a reward or a punishment. You should both be in a playful, exploring frame of mind; this is about building a foundation for your mutual fantasy, rather than being a fantasy itself. Relax and let go of any particular goal; just enjoy the sensuality and intimacy of what you are doing.

If it helps, think of it as a rehearsal.

Take your time as you spank, paddle or whip him. Keep him aroused and encourage him to ask for breaks. Try doing something unexpected during these breaks. For example: kissing him soundly; letting him kiss your feet; offering him a comforting, sympathetic embrace; making him hold your riding crop between his teeth for a while; applying a cooling oil or lotion to his skin. Get him to tell you how these break activities make him feel. Or, ask him what he'd like to happen. You might discover some previously unknown submissive response that you'll enjoy triggering later...

This is mainly about you exploring and inflicting sensations and experiences on him. There will be plenty of opportunities for him to repay your attentions on another occasion.

Stay away from harsh sensations, particularly in the early stages. Experiment with multiple repetitions of a lighter stroke, instead of just assuming you should progress from light blows to heavier ones; a very light tap, rapidly delivered to the same point time after time, can eventually have a more powerful effect than a single heavy blow.

Each time you cause him some new sensation, have him tell

you the intensity of what he feels on a scale of 1-10, where 1 indicates the mildest sensation and 10 indicates that he needs you to stop. If you prefer him not to speak, arrange him on his hands and knees and have him signal silently with his fingers: all fingers hidden = "everything is okay"; ten fingers spread out = "Ouch!".

Build slowly, allowing him time for reflection and anticipation. Unless you and he are into "boundary pushing", try to avoid reaching 10. The aim is to understand how the force, timing and nature of your blows corresponds to his ability to tolerate them. With practice, you should gain a much greater insight into the sensations you are inflicting on your man.

For the opposite effect of the cooling oils or lotions mentioned above, try a warming oil such as peppermint; use these carefully on healthy skin only (never on broken skin or mucus membrane), and be aware that these will greatly enhance his sensitivity should you continue with further discipline after using them. Until you have gained experience and trust, it is better to reserve warming oils for the final touch.

Throughout this exercise, make sure your man understands the purpose of what you are doing together, and that he is to be honest with you about how the sensations and intensities change depending on what you do. He needs to remember that knowledge is power and that his honesty is an empowering gift. This is not the time for him to be macho.

Going through a discipline-based learning experience like this can uncover new things, and thus have a strong emotional effect on both you and him. Afterward, take whatever together-time you both need for mutual comfort, reassurance and recovery. The same goes for any session that is particularly powerful or draining for either of you.

Week 28: Pussy Slam

While you are making love in the missionary position and he's busy kissing your face or upper body, put your hands on his head or shoulders and push him down forcefully, bringing his mouth into position between your legs.

Have him stay where you've put him while he pleasures you orally. Hold his head in place if you wish. Keep him in position for as long as you like.

Week 29: Exercise Program

If your man isn't in as good a physical shape as you'd prefer, get him started on a physical training program aimed at improving his physique and fitness: push-ups, sit-ups, dumb-bells, weights, squats, exercise bike, running, whatever you feel would benefit him most. Have him research and design a suitable schedule.

If you have any doubts because of his current physical condition or age, seek medical advice first. Participate if/when you like, with a riding crop in hand for "motivation".

Once he's made a start, bring some exercise routines into your bedroom: have him "perform" for you, or have him do push-ups while you recline with outstretched legs so that he can kiss your feet between presses (making him hold position until he has worshipped your feet properly provides a way of challenging him, once he's strong enough to handle it). Adapt to other kinds of exercises as you wish. For example, he could kiss the tip of your suitably-proffered riding crop at the highest point of each sit-up.

Once he's done, consider a reward in keeping with the activity. For example, give him a few strokes of the riding crop he's been kissing.

Week 30: Exercise Program, Reversed

If you want to get in better shape, make him serve as your personal trainer, pushing and exhorting you to work harder. Make it clear that he is responsible for motivating you and getting you into shape.

This one is good if you want to bring out the strong side of your man. It could even develop into a full "switch" (where he expresses his dominant side and you express your submissive one) if you and he are that way inclined. If that's not what you want, make it very clear to him before you begin that you will have the final word at all times; his role is to encourage and persuade, not to compel.

If it is what you want, then make sure he gets the message. Some subtle (or even not-so-subtle) hints might be in order…

Week 31: Secret Dress Code

Send him out into the world inappropriately (secretly) dressed. For example, make him wear a cock ring, or no underclothes. Or, dress him in panties or pantyhose or some other hidden feminine garment of your choice.

Have him text you every hour confirming that he is still wearing the items concerned.

At the end of the day, make him strip in front of you to show what he has been wearing. Judge his performance. Did he miss any text messages? Is everything in place as it should be? Are any garments stretched, stained or laddered?

Make him explain any shortcomings. If he has a reasonable excuse, punish him. If not, express your displeasure and do not reward him with any femdom play for a suitable period (at the very least, the rest of that evening). If he performed well, permit him to please you with his mouth or grant some other reward of your choice.

August-September: Weeks 32-35

Week 32: Mystery Assignation

Book a double room in a hotel (make sure you get two key cards).
Have a drink with him in the bar and then send him up to the room
alone. He is to put the "Do Not Disturb" sign on the door and
then get undressed, showered and groomed. Finally, he is to put
on a blindfold and wait. Tell him that you have something unusual
planned for him, without specifying what that is.

After a suitable interval, join him. Check that his blindfold is
secure. Don't say anything (except maybe "Shhhh!!!", if he speaks)
but have your way with him. Maybe be rougher or more forceful
than usual. Arrange to be wearing a different perfume or clothes
that are unfamiliar to him, if you wish. Wearing a sexy mask will
also help preserve the fantasy in the event his blindfold slips (to
avoid this risk, you might want to fit him with a hood instead of a
blindfold).

If he speaks out of turn, particularly if he tries to get you to
speak, punish him.

If you wish to add a final flourish, leave without saying a word
and then return a few minutes later, as if you've only just come up
from the bar.

Week 33: Sexy Story Time

Choose an erotic story or novel that you think will appeal to both
of you. It should be one that follows the experiences of a submissive male. Have your man start reading it out loud for you. Encourage him to invent and perform different voices to represent the
various characters. Let him know how well or badly he is doing,
and what the consequences will be if you don't think he's trying
hard enough.

Take the part of narrator yourself if you enjoy reading out loud to him. Or switch back and forward, with each of you reading a chapter and then handing the book over. It's your choice.

Whenever the story takes a kinky turn, consider taking a short break from reading while you inflict something comparable on your man.

Whenever the fictional male performs some erotic service or favour for his lover or Mistress, ditto.

Fantasy erotica often includes extreme or risky activities, so tone thing down as necessary to stay safe. The idea is to create your own experience based on the story, not to follow it slavishly. Also, there's no need to finish the story in a single sitting. You might want to split a novel-length story over several days or even weeks.

Variation 1: Feminising/Cross-Dressing Version. Read a sexy story just as before, but choose one where the central character is a submissive woman. Your man is to experience, as closely as possible, what this character goes through. Substitute appropriately (keeping things as similar to the story as you can manage) where the gender of the character makes it impossible to perform the same activities with your man.

Variation 2: You won't always be in the mood to put the story aside; nor is every fictional event suited to being brought to life on the spot. So keep a notebook handy and write down things you'd like to do later, when you're in the mood or the opportunity presents itself. Don't let him see what you are writing; the fact that you are privately taking notes is a potent demonstration of your female authority.

Week 34: A Subtle Sign

Pre-arrange a silent signal to command some submissive service from your man. This can be used in private, in which case the service may be due immediately, or in public, in which case you are informing him that you expect it later.

Examples:

- Let your index finger and middle finger represent your legs. Press the cleft between the fingers to his mouth — he is to go down on you.
- Press the corresponding two fingertips to his mouth — he is to worship your feet.
- As above, but then slide your fingers along his lips — he is to start at your feet and work his way up.
- Loosen his tie, shirt button or some other item of clothing — he is to strip for you.
- Stroke his throat — he's to fetch his collar, and put it in if you permit him to do this himself.
- Tap your fingers across the back of his hand — he's to fetch your whip.

The above are all hand-signals but you can arrange any non-verbal method of communication you choose.

When communicating in public, you may also wish to pre-arrange some way in which he can privately indicate his understanding and acceptance of your message.

If he misses a sign or forgets to respond to it, inflict some punishment. You don't have to tell him that he missed it; let him work it out for himself (and do his best to make up for his mistake).

Week 35: Permission to Come

Train him to ask for your permission before he has an orgasm.

Assign a ritual form of words that he must use, for example, "Please may I come, Mistress?"

He is to use this before allowing himself to ejaculate (unless you have previously made it clear this rule has been relaxed).

Variation: Train him to take the ritual further depending on the answer you make. For example:

- If you answer "Yes", he may come when he is ready.
- If you answer "Five" (or some other number) then he is to come within that many strokes or thrusts. If he doesn't get there in time, he misses his orgasm.
- If you answer "Maybe", the current activity continues. At some point, you may change your answer, giving him the opportunity to come. He is not to ask again.
- If you answer "Not yet", the current activity continues. He may ask again.
- If you answer "No", you're indicating that whatever you are doing will continue for as long as you wish, but he should resign himself to being left frustrated at the end.

You may find it more satisfying to restrict yourself to two or three answers, in order to focus your authority on those specific areas. It's up to you.

September-October: Weeks 36-39

Week 36: Breakfast in Bed

Before you both sleep after some night-time scenario that has left your man chaste and frustrated, inform him that he is to bring you breakfast in bed the next morning. Tell him what you would prefer and what time you require it to be served. He is to wake early, prepare your tray as ordered, and serve it to you in bed. Have him do this while naked and/or collared, if you wish to further indulge his submissive nature.

If you enjoy this kind of service and decide to command it regularly, consider acquiring a special bed-table (which is essentially a tray with legs, designed to be used as you recline in bed). If he is a decent craftsman, creating such an offering could make an ideal project for him to exercise his skills.

He should clear everything away after you have eaten your breakfast. If you still have an appetite, summon him back into bed and allow him to eat his. Or if you are feeling particularly indulgent, allow him to relieve his frustration from the night before by having intercourse with you to the point of orgasm.

Week 37: As Good as the Real Thing?

Use (or have your man use) a commercial penis-casting kit to make a dildo in the shape of his penis. Be as involved as you wish.

(Whoever buys and uses the kit should do their research. Read online reviews from previous purchasers. The instructions that come with these kits must be followed very carefully.)

When it's ready, lube it up and use it for your own pleasure, then make him lick it clean. Or, make him "fellate" his own penis while you watch. If penetrating him anally is part of your routine, use it for that too if you like. The usual hygiene considerations apply.

Week 38: Cruel and Unusual

Occasionally you may wish to inflict an erotic punishment that is harsher than usual.

(Depending on how masochistic your man is, a harsher punishment might equate to a greater reward).

Anal Hook: This is a sex toy designed to be inserted anally, and then secured by rope or chain to some fastening point. If you link it to his collar by a short enough leash, you can compel him to keep his back nicely arched. If you spank or paddle your man in this state, his inability to make the slightest gesture of self-protection will increase his sense of vulnerability to the maximum. Of course, you will also be denied the visual feedback that his body language usually gives you, so proceed with care and only after you have gained experience of how he responds to corporal punishment.

An anal hook with a ball on the end is more intimidating than a plain one, and lends itself to slow, ritual insertion; a plain, smooth hook is easier to insert and thus more practical. Use plenty of lube in either case.

Chastisement in Chastity: Subjecting him to a spanking or paddling while he's locked into a chastity device prevents him from becoming fully aroused by the erotic aspect of his punishment, making the experience harder for him to endure. Frequent pauses to tease him through (and around) the device will help keep him as physically aroused as he can be in that situation.

Take care not to inadvertently overdo it — if he becomes completely flaccid then the erotic aspect of his punishment will no longer exist. Don't go to that extreme unless you intend to do so, and have his consent.

Week 39: Towers of Hanoi

Set up a "Towers of Hanoi" game in your bedroom. If you and your man are not familiar with solving this puzzle, which involves moving differently-sized rings from one post to another, you will find plenty of guidance online.

All the rings start on the left hand post; move them to the right hand post according to the rules of the game.

Define when a ring is to be moved: one a day, perhaps, plus an extra one when he does something in particular to please you. When he displeases you, you may wish to move a ring back. When all the rings have moved to the final post, he is eligible for an orgasm (or some other reward, if you do not wish to use this as a male chastity counter).

Choose the number of rings depending on how many days you want the puzzle to last. Three rings will take seven days to move, if one is moved correctly each day. Four rings will take fifteen days while five rings will take 31 days, so you have a natural way to aim for a week, a fortnight or a month.

Some rituals and embellishments to consider:

- Make him clear the game when it completes.
- Make him move the ring each day, or when he has earned a reward.
- Make him make a wrong (delaying) move when he has earned a punishment.
- Leave an object such as your whip lying across the game to indicate that he is not to touch it that day.
- When the puzzle nears completion, offer him the choice of some other deeply-desired reward or punishment ... but at the price of clearing the game back to its start.
- Take responsibility for the game yourself; forbid him to touch it at all.

October - November: Weeks 40-44

Week 40: Punishment List

Draw up a list of possible punishments for your man.

Try not to limit yourself to obvious ones like paddling, spanking and whipping. Here are some examples to help get your imagination going; use them as the starting point for a list that's specific to you and your man.

Corner Time — he is to spend a specified period reflecting on his behavior as he stands facing into a corner — naked, if you choose.

Cold Shower — he is to strip off and get under the cold running shower, remaining there for however long you say (set a timer if you like). This becomes intolerable more quickly than you might imagine; try ducking into and out of a cold shower yourself to understand what impact a more extended shower would have.

Letter of Apology — he is to write a letter to you, apologizing for whatever he did wrong and explaining what he will do to improve his behavior in future.

Solitary Confinement — he is to remain in a particular room for however long you say. This is similar to corner time except that he can use the confinement constructively, perhaps even correcting whatever fault led to the punishment in the first place.

Loss of Privilege — deny him something that is not vital to his wellbeing, but that he enjoys or has come to expect. Does he naturally expect to sit next to you on the couch, beer in hand, while you watch a movie together? If you need to teach him a lesson, how about putting him at your feet with a glass of water instead?

Loss of Privacy — set a period in which he is not allowed to close any door in your home unless he has your dispensation to do so. Lacking that permission, he is to leave the door ajar.

Unpleasant Chore — every home has unpleasant or awkward

chores that get put off because nobody wants to do them ... cleaning the oven, scrubbing the shower base, getting the gunk off the barbecue, defrosting the freezer, washing or detailing the car ... these can make perfect punishment tasks where your man can make amends while also learning to mend his ways.

Have him draw up his own list, ranking punishments that arouse him (maybe secretly) down to punishments he would genuinely hate. He is to give his completed list to you. While there's no reason to treat it as a "To Do" list (he is not the one in charge, after all!) it can still give you valuable insights and ideas.

If you like, sit down with him to compare the two lists. Is his list too short, or missing a punishment you particularly liked? You could make something of that, if you wished!

Variation: Make him nominate one punishment from the lists that he wishes never to be applied. What would he be prepared to do to gain temporary immunity from that punishment?

Week 41: Getting Better at Going Down

Have him research online sources and books for exercises and techniques that will help him improve his cunnilingus technique. He is to devise an exercise program and follow it to your satisfaction.

Offer positive feedback as he progresses; let him know that you value his efforts.

Don't be shy about helping and guiding him if that's what it takes to make his tongue really dance for you; a submissive male craves this and should not see his manhood being undermined by constructive criticism from his Mistress. Only you can know what will be most helpful to your slave in this regard, but where femdom is concerned it's often the case that the stricter the teacher, the more memorable the lesson.

Week 42: Toy Box

Make him prepare a place for you to keep your whips and toys.

If he's a competent craftsman, he can make a lockable box or chest or adapt an existing one. If not, at least have him put up some hooks and/or shelves in a suitable discreet place.

Instruct him to put your toys away in their new home. He must follow any rituals you have created while doing this (for example, when putting away your whips, you may decide that he is only hold them by "his" end rather than the handle, which naturally belongs to you).

When he's done, inspect his work and offer your appreciation or constructive criticism. If you need to criticise, be fair but strict. If you feel a punishment is appropriate, apply it and then make him re-do the work that fell short of your required standard.

Finally, if the box is lockable, have him kneel while he presents you with the key.

Week 43: Piercing

If you're interested in this then ear-piercing is a good place to begin; the earring can become symbolic of your ownership. Arranging for a female practitioner to perform the piercing can have symbolic power, too.

Later you may wish to move on to other body parts. Both of you should do your research, including on healing times and care requirements, before committing to anything.

A penis piercing is perhaps the most intimate sign of owner-ship, and is particularly effective if you are into chastity play. A de-termined male may demonstrate a surprising ability to escape from a device that simply locks around his genitals; locking it to a pierc-ing is much more secure.

Always use a licensed practitioner and make sure your slave is educated about how to care for any piercing he undergoes. When arranging a chastity piercing, the practitioner **must** be informed of the intended use.

Week 44: Dildo Play

Make him please you with a dildo or vibrator while being denied any pleasure himself. Or, please yourself while making him watch; restrain him if you like.

Variation 1: Have intercourse with him while he's wearing a strap-on (his penis being locked into a chastity device) so that he has the experience of love-making while being denied any direct genital sensation.

Variation 2: Enjoy him while he's strapped into a "dildo gag" (this is essentially a gag that buckles around his head, with a dildo projecting outward from his mouth).

November - December: Weeks 45-48

Week 45: Mark Your Man

Mark your man to identify him as your property.

Unless you and he are already comfortable with tattooing, you'll want to start with something durable but not permanent. It's not uncommon for people to write on their own skin with a ball point, sharpie or even a marking pen occasionally, but since you can't be sure what is in the ink, it's not something you want to do too frequently or in large amounts. As a one off, though, writing *"Property of Mistress ... "* on a discreet part of his body with a ballpoint pen could be a sexy way to lay your first written claim on your willing slave.

For more regular but non-permanent use, consider henna tattoos. These are available in in kit form, can last a week or more, and can be renewed as they start to fade. Natural henna is plant-based and very safe, but ensure you buy from a reputable supplier and if in doubt about possible allergies, test on a small area first.

To ink a permanent mark you'll need to involve a qualified tattoo artist. As a caring Mistress, you must only do this when you have considered your man's long-term welfare. It can seem unromantic to consider such things, but a tattoo with a lover's name can be regretted years or decades later — and not necessarily through either person's fault. The caring, communicating couple will talk things through and handle the matter through informed, self-aware consent.

Week 46: Is He Sitting Comfortably?

Make him wear a butt plug while you're out together on a date or social event.

For extra spice, use a plug incorporating a vibrator that's remotely controlled. If money's no object and you want to demonstrate your power and control over him while you're apart, consider a Bluetooth-controlled vibrating plug that can be activated by a smartphone app.

Week 47: Class Action

You will take on the role of a sexy teacher from the days when corporal punishment was a commonplace form of school discipline, while he will be your pupil. If both of you are in costumes (you in something sexy but severe, him in "school uniform") then it will help make the fantasy more real.

Assign him some school work on which he will be tested. For example, have him learn a poem that he will be expected to recite from memory while you check his performance from your own copy. Allow at least a few days so that you can build anticipation (this will increase the impact of the event itself).

Arrange the time and place at which he will be expected to perform. Ideally, have him sit at an improvised school desk while you stand before him. If you and he are into making kinky recordings, set up a camera to record his performance and any punishment he receives ... the presence of the camera can add to the fun (and his sense of vulnerability) even if you secretly plan to delete the movie afterwards.

When the time comes, have him recite the poem. Whenever he makes a mistake or stumbles over the words, he receives a stroke across his palm and has to remove part of his "school uniform".

(If you don't want to use a poem, assign something else that will work in the same way. One possibility is to have him study for a test or quiz to be completed verbally "in class").

Once he is naked, if he makes another mistake, he will receive a stroke across his buttocks instead.

If he makes no mistakes, reward him in some way. Maybe he'll be invited into Miss's apartment and up to her bedroom … or maybe he'll be chastised for being a little too pleased with himself!

A traditional instrument of punishment in British and Irish schools was the tawse or leather strap, which is recommended for this fantasy. If you are confident that you can safely handle a harsher instrument such as a cane, you might use that instead; it has a similar historical resonance. You could also use a paddle or riding crop if you prefer, but these are less in keeping with the school discipline fantasy.

Week 48: Anal Play

Indulge in some anal play with him, if the idea appeals to you.

Always make sure the person receiving anal attention is scrupulously clean first. Keep a plastic bowl or bucket handy, to drop any toys into so he can clean and sterilize them later. Spread an old towel on areas that might get messed up. Use latex gloves if you like and if neither of you are allergic.

If the idea of such precautions squicks you out too much, non-penetrative anal play might suit you better — or you might prefer to avoid this area altogether.

Assuming that's not the case…

Pegging: penetrate him with a strap-on, or just use a dildo. Use plenty of lube, go slowly, and combine twisting with thrusting to get things moving. This can be a degrading and feminizing experience for a man. It can also be highly stimulating for him, while also allowing you to experience a sense of erotic power that you won't find in any other way.

Anilingus: have him orally worship your anus. For the sake of your vaginal health, get any pussy worship out of the way before you let him go to work on your ass and/or institute a rigorous Oral Inspection and cleansing regime as part of your regular femdom activities.

Squeaky Clean: have him cleanse himself with an enema (he must purchase suitable equipment) according to your schedule — before you play, every day, it's up to you. He should research the subject to learn how to perform this cleansing safely and effectively. Anybody using enemas should inform themselves of possible adverse effects and how to avoid them.

December: Weeks 49-52

Week 49: Ritual of Love

When you make love, begin with extended foreplay. Make sure you get whatever stimulation you need short of intercourse: take advantage of his hands, his mouth, his penis as long as there's no vaginal penetration. In short, enjoy whatever body parts you wish and reciprocate as desired.

When you're ready for the initial phase of intercourse, adopt an on-top position. Tie his hands to the headboard, if you like. The only rule here is that he is not allowed to come. Treat him as your personal living sex toy. There's no need to restrict yourself to pussy-penis contact at this stage; his mouth is right there too.

For the final phase, untie him and allow him on top. Proceed with missionary-position sex, but keep things slow for as long as you please. Don't allow him to speed up and climax until you give the signal by reaching around and spanking or paddling his rump.

Variation: Train him to go wild on you with his penis, hands and mouth when you reach around to deliver a single spank, but to back off before he ejaculates. Enjoy him in this way as many times as you desire, then signal that he's allowed to come with several hard spanks in succession.

Week 50: Mistress's Slave Girl

If you feel the need to temper your own dominance with submission, or if you simply wish to step away from the Mistress persona from time to time, create the role of a seductive slave girl who is occasionally sent by your other (Mistress) persona to prepare the male slave for Mistress's later attentions, or to reward him for his service, or to celebrate his birthday etc.

Wear a sexy mask and/or costume if you wish, to differentiate the roles.

Bringing this second role into play can free you to attend to him in ways that you might not feel appropriate for your Mistress persona.

Week 51: Sexy Scrunchies

Claim his genitals as your intimate property by trapping them with something that is also intimately yours.

You'll need an old hair scrunchie or a similar loop of elasticized material. If you wear tights, cutting across the legs of an old pair will produce suitably stretchy rings. Choose an unglamorous knitted pair whose fabric will remain forgiving to sensitive skin even when under some pressure.

Start by encircling the base of his genitals (next to his body) and then make another loop around his scrotum so that his balls are trapped too. Using elasticized fabric makes it easy to arrange things snugly without them being over-tight. Always leave enough play in the elastic so that it will be easy to remove later.

Use a second scrunchie/loop if one alone isn't big enough, or if you want to bind him more thoroughly by adding several layers.

A snug loop around the base of his genitals will make it harder for him to control (delay) his orgasm, while the loop trapping his balls will place them entirely at the mercy of your squeezing fingers; he will thus be rendered extremely vulnerable. If you play up the "cruel" side of your nature, he might even feel a little scared!

If you want to make it harder for him to come, try placing a snug loop around the base of just his penis. If the elasticized loops get messed up with lube or body fluids, it's his job to clean them later.

Variation: Practice capturing his balls with your hand alone so that you can claim him in this way whenever you like. Encircle his scrotum with your forefinger and thumb so as to trap his testicles, then use your other fingers to let him know how completely he's in your power. You might find this awkward at first, particularly if you have small hands, but it gets easier with practice. In the meantime, you could inform him that he's to prepare himself with an elasticized ring as described above, each time he presents himself for your enjoyment.

Week 52: New Year, New Skill

Instruct your man to learn a new domestic or household skill. This could be something you usually handle, something you'd normally pay for, or perhaps even something completely new that you'd like to bring into your life. How about…

- making your favorite cocktail
- preparing from scratch some gourmet or artisan food that you would normally buy ready-made
- doing the weekly laundry
- hand-washing of your delicate lingerie
- ironing your blouses
- something entirely new and creative?

Where appropriate, be prepared to spend some time teaching him how you like the chore or task done.

You can create additional pressure and motivation by setting a time limit. If he fails to master the skill in time, assign an appropriate punishment.

Once he's learned, have him use his new skill. If it's something you usually do, he could take it over in future. Playful nit-picking and punishment is appropriate if desired, but as long as your man has made a good effort, make sure he knows deep down that you're pleased with him and value his work.

Variation: Instead of making him learn some new domestic skill, consider having him do something that he's already good at, making sure it's not directly to do with his erotic and romantic relationship with you.

Try for something practical rather than intellectual; he can write you a sonnet another time. Instead, have him use his craftsmanship, inventiveness, strength, or other workmanlike skills on your behalf. Even if he's not particularly competent at things like laundry or ironing, his diligence and ability for hard work can be of great value — in the coming year will you have a flower bed that needs digging, a lawn that needs cutting, a wall that needs painting?

Tell him that you expect him to use the chosen skill for your benefit, and that it's up to him to show you what he can do. Warn him not to disappoint you, while also hinting that a good performance will not be overlooked.

You can let him choose what to do or direct his efforts as you please. Then sit back and enjoy the results. Show your appreciation through suitable rewards and/or punishments.

Other Femdom Titles by Lucy Fairbourne

Femdom Guides

Femdom for Nice Girls:
A Self-Guided Manual for the Caring Mistress

From childhood onwards, females are encouraged into subservient roles, so that taking the lead can feel strange and unnatural, even "unfeminine" and "not nice". We are discouraged from aggressively grabbing what we want, and instead encouraged to sacrifice and nurture. We are taught to be prizes, not competitors.

Surely, there has to be more to life than that. Many men — the ones who value assertiveness (and even a little cruelty) in their female lovers would agree. So would many women.

If you're one of these women, or if your man is one of those men, then this book could be just what you and he have been searching for.

Male Chastity:
A Guide for Keyholders

A non-threatening, female-friendly introduction to the topic of male chastity, ideal for nervous keyholders, beginning femdoms, or as a love-offering from a would-be-chastened male.

Femdom Stories

No Safe Words

Struggling to come to terms with his own submissive nature, Matthew has rebelled against Marie-Laure's loving authority, only to find he needs her female domination more than he ever knew. How far will he go to prove he is worthy of another chance with her? More to the point, how far will she require him to go before she'll consider taking him back?

Just Dessert

When middle-aged Frank spots the beautiful young Orianne in a chic Paris hotel, there's nothing that Ellie, his long-suffering wife, can say or do to make him behave himself. Little does he know that Orianne is the bait for an elaborate scam intended to cost him almost everything. How could he? Even Orianne is in the dark about the real intentions of her brilliant but devious mentor, Madame Claire Cheron.

Lightning Source UK Ltd.
Milton Keynes UK
UKHW010624131221
395525UK00001B/195